TYPE 2 DIABETES COOKBOOK FOR BEGINNERS

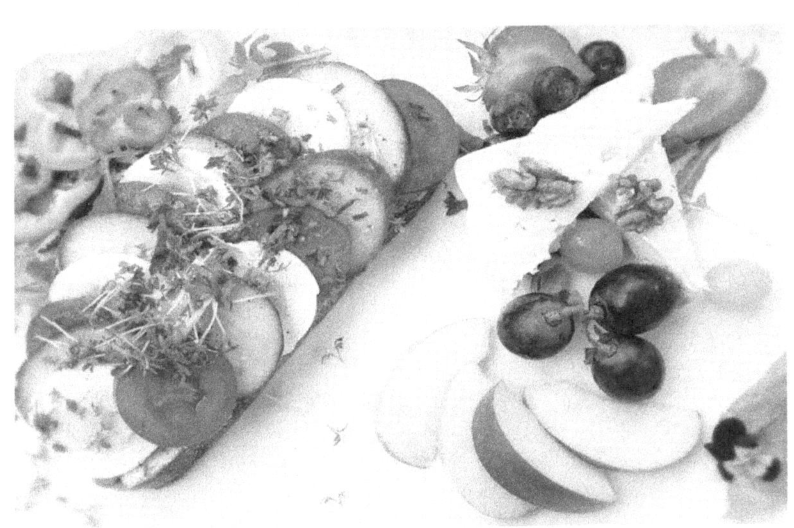

NATURALLY CONTROL BLOOD SUGAR AND ACHIEVE AN A1C BELOW 5.7% SIMPLE, DELICIOUS RECIPES FOR RECLAIMING YOUR HEALTH

DEBBIE G BERGERON

COPYRIGHT AND DISCLAIMER

Copyright © 2024 Debbie G Bergeron. All rights reserved.

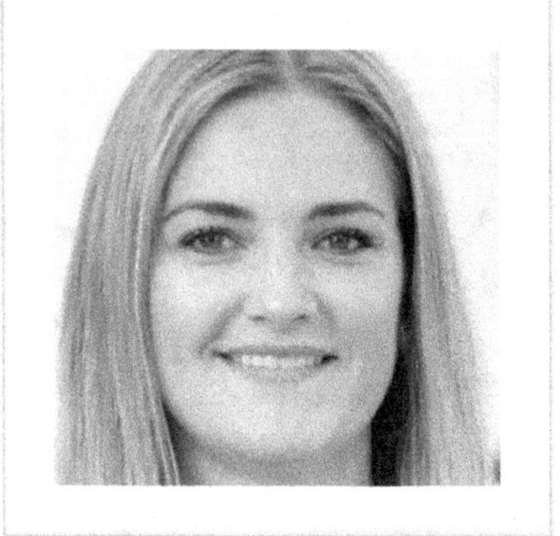

Notice of Disclaimer

This book contains material that should only be used for educational and informative reasons; it is not meant to be used as medical advice. The information is based on the author's own research, experience, and understanding of diet and diabetes care. Despite every attempt to guarantee its correctness, the material is not a replacement for expert medical advice, diagnosis, or treatment.

Asking your doctor or another trained health expert for guidance on any medical issue or dietary changes is always a beneficial idea. Never ignore medical advice from professionals or put off getting it because of anything you've read in this book.

Any negative effects or repercussions arising from using the recipes, advice, or ideas in this book are not the responsibility of the author or publisher. The efficacy of any health or nutrition plan is dependent on a variety of individual circumstances; therefore, individual outcomes may differ.

ABOUT THE AUTHOR

Debbie G. Bergeron is a chef specialist with a focus on diabetes friendly food and a fervent supporter of healthy living. With a background in nutrition and a personal path that has brought her close to the field of diabetes treatment, Debbie has made it her mission to use food's power to empower others to live better, more balanced lives.

Professional Experience:

Debbie has over ten years of experience working as a registered nutritionist and dietitian. She has a degree in nutrition and dietetics. She has cultivated tight relationships with customers to create customized meal plans that address a range of nutritional requirements, especially for individuals with type 2 diabetes. In order to encourage nutritional practices that are both enjoyable and sustainable, she has worked with wellness initiatives, diabetes educators, and healthcare professionals.

Personal Story: Debbie's dedication to diabetic friendly cuisine stems from her own family's diabetes struggles. After seeing the struggles loved ones experience, she has made it her goal to develop delectable and approachable dishes that make controlling diabetes more pleasurable. Her professional knowledge and life experiences combine to provide thoughtful, tasty diabetic control advice.

Debbie's culinary philosophy is that flavour should never be sacrificed for the sake of health. Her cooking approach is based on using whole, fresh foods to produce dishes that are not only flavorful but also nutrient dense. She works to make healthy cooking accessible to everyone and stresses the value of balance, portion management, and mindful eating.

journals and media: Debbie is a prolific writer who has written for many health and wellness journals in addition to her profession as a nutritionist. She has shared her knowledge of healthy cuisine and diabetes care in a number of media venues. She is a sought after speaker and consultant in the sector because of her kind demeanour and useful advice.

Debbie's aim is to enable people to take charge of their health by making educated food choices and to provide them the resources and skills they need to succeed in the long run. She keeps creating new recipes, teaching resources, and supporting networks to help people navigate the challenges of managing their diabetes.

Debbie G. Bergeron is committed to helping people achieve and enjoy healthy living, and she looks forward to supporting and motivating you on your path to improved health.

TABLE OF CONTENTS

INTRODUCTION

Welcome to a new chapter in your health journey! Whether you've recently been diagnosed with Type 2 diabetes or have been managing it for some time, this book is designed to be your trusted companion in the kitchen. "Type 2 Diabetes Cookbook for Beginners: Naturally Control Blood Sugar and Achieve an A1C Below 5.7% Simple, Delicious Recipes for Reclaiming Your Health" is more than just a collection of recipes; it's a guide to transforming your diet, your habits, and your life.

Welcome to Your New Healthy Life

Embarking on a journey to better health can be both exciting and daunting. This book aims to make that journey as smooth and enjoyable as possible. By incorporating delicious, easy to make recipes into your daily routine, you'll discover that managing Type 2 diabetes doesn't have to mean giving up the foods you love. Instead, it's about finding new, healthier ways to enjoy your meals and improve your overall wellbeing.

Understanding Type 2 Diabetes

Type 2 diabetes is a chronic condition that affects how your body metabolizes sugar (glucose). It's characterized by insulin resistance and impaired insulin secretion, leading to elevated blood glucose levels. Understanding the nature of Type 2 diabetes is crucial for effective management and prevention. Here's a comprehensive overview:

What is Type 2 Diabetes?

Insulin Resistance: In Type 2 diabetes, the body's cells become resistant to insulin, a hormone that helps glucose enter cells from the bloodstream. As a result, glucose builds up in the blood.

Impaired Insulin Production: Over time, the pancreas may not produce enough insulin to keep blood glucose levels within a normal range.

Risk Factors

Several factors can increase the risk of developing Type 2 diabetes, including:

Genetics: A family history of diabetes can increase your risk.

Age: The risk increases with age, particularly after 45.

Obesity: Excess body fat, especially around the abdomen, is a major risk factor.

Physical Inactivity: A sedentary lifestyle contributes to weight gain and insulin resistance.

Unhealthy Diet: Diets high in refined carbohydrates, added sugars, and unhealthy fats can increase risk.

Ethnicity: Certain ethnic groups, including African American, Hispanic, Native American, and Asian American populations, are at higher risk.

Gestational Diabetes: Women who had gestational diabetes during pregnancy are at a higher risk of developing Type 2 diabetes later.

Symptoms

- Type 2 diabetes often develops slowly, and symptoms may be subtle. Common signs include:
- Increased Thirst and Frequent Urination: Excess glucose in the blood draws water from tissues, leading to dehydration and frequent urination.

- **Fatigue:** The body's inability to efficiently use glucose for energy can cause persistent tiredness.

- Blurred Vision: High blood sugar levels can cause fluid to be pulled from the lenses of the eyes, affecting vision.

- Slow Healing Sores or Frequent Infections: High blood glucose levels can impair the body's ability to heal wounds and fight infections.

- Unexplained Weight Loss or Gain: Weight loss can occur when the body starts breaking down muscle and fat for energy. Conversely, weight gain can result from insulin resistance and overeating.

Diagnosis

Type 2 diabetes is diagnosed through blood tests that measure blood glucose levels. Common tests include:

- Fasting Plasma Glucose (FPG) Test: Measures blood glucose after an overnight fast.

- Oral Glucose Tolerance Test (OGTT): Measures blood glucose levels after fasting and then drinking a glucose rich beverage.

- Hemoglobin A1c Test: Provides an average blood glucose level over the past 23 months.

Complications

If not managed properly, Type 2 diabetes can lead to serious complications:

Cardiovascular Disease: Increased risk of heart disease and stroke.

Neuropathy: Nerve damage, often leading to pain, numbness, or tingling in the extremities.

Nephropathy: Kidney damage that can lead to kidney failure.

Retinopathy: Eye damage that can result in vision loss.

Foot Problems: Poor blood flow and nerve damage can lead to infections and ulcers.

Management and Treatment

Managing Type 2 diabetes involves a combination of lifestyle changes, medication, and monitoring:

- Diet: Adopting a balanced, nutrient dense diet that controls carbohydrate intake and supports overall health.
- Exercise: Regular physical activity helps improve insulin sensitivity and aids in weight management.
- Medication: Oral medications or insulin may be prescribed to help manage blood glucose levels.

- Monitoring: Regular monitoring of blood glucose levels to ensure they stay within target ranges.
- Education and Support: Working with healthcare professionals and support groups to manage the condition effectively.

Prevention

Preventing Type 2 diabetes involves making lifestyle changes that reduce risk factors:

Maintain a Healthy Weight: Achieving and maintaining a healthy weight through diet and exercise.

Be Physically Active: Engage in regular physical activity, aiming for at least 150 minutes of moderate exercise per week.

Healthy Eating: Follow a diet rich in fruits, vegetables, whole grains, and lean proteins while limiting processed foods and sugary beverages.

Regular Check Ups: Monitor blood glucose levels and undergo regular health screenings.

The Role of Diet in Managing Diabetes

Effective management of diabetes is largely influenced by dietary choices. Understanding the role of diet in diabetes management is crucial for maintaining blood glucose levels within target ranges and reducing the risk of complications.

Understanding Carbohydrates

Carbohydrates have the most significant impact on blood sugar levels. When you consume carbohydrates, they are broken down into glucose, which enters the bloodstream and raises blood sugar levels. Managing carbohydrate intake is essential for controlling blood glucose levels.

Choose Low Glycemic Index Foods: Foods with a low glycemic index (GI) release glucose slowly into the bloodstream, which helps maintain steady blood sugar levels. Examples include whole grains, legumes, and non-starchy vegetables.

Monitor Portion Sizes: Even healthy carbohydrates can impact blood sugar if consumed in large quantities. Use portion control to manage your carbohydrate intake effectively.

Incorporating Fiber

Fiber is a type of carbohydrate that doesn't raise blood sugar levels. It helps slow the absorption of glucose and promotes digestive health.

Opt for High Fiber Foods: Include plenty of fruits, vegetables, legumes, and whole grains in your diet. Fiber helps with blood sugar control and can improve overall glycemic control.

Balancing Protein and Fat

Protein and fats have minimal impact on blood sugar levels, but they are essential for a balanced diet.

Include Lean Proteins: Incorporate lean meats, poultry, fish, tofu, and legumes into your meals. Protein helps with muscle maintenance and repair, and it can help you feel full and satisfied.

Choose Healthy Fats: Focus on sources of unsaturated fats such as avocados, nuts, seeds, and olive oil. Limit saturated and trans fats, which can contribute to heart disease.

Monitoring Portion Sizes

Portion control is important for managing blood glucose levels and overall calorie intake.

Consuming large portions, even of healthy foods, can lead to weight gain and difficulties in blood sugar control.

Use Portion Guides: Utilize measuring cups, a food scale, or visual portion guides to help keep portions in check.

Regular Meal Timing

Eating at regular intervals helps maintain steady blood sugar levels. Skipping meals can lead to fluctuations in blood sugar levels, making it harder to manage diabetes.

Plan Balanced Meals: Aim for three main meals and healthy snacks if needed. Each meal should include a balance of carbohydrates, protein, and fats.

Reducing Added Sugars and Refined Carbs

Added sugars and refined carbohydrates can cause rapid spikes in blood glucose levels and provide little nutritional value.

Read Food Labels: Avoid foods high in added sugars and refined carbs such as sugary beverages, sweets, and white bread. Opt for whole foods and minimally processed options.

Staying Hydrated

Adequate hydration supports overall health and helps regulate blood sugar levels.

Drink Plenty of Water: Aim for 810 glasses of water a day. Avoid sugary drinks and limit consumption of caffeinated beverages.

Personalized Dietary Plans

Individual needs can vary based on factors such as age, weight, activity level, and specific health conditions.

Consult a Healthcare Professional: Work with a registered dietitian or healthcare provider to create a personalized dietary plan that meets your specific needs and health goals.

HOW TO USE THIS COOKBOOK

Welcome to "Type 2 Diabetes Cookbook for Beginners: Naturally Control Blood Sugar and Achieve an A1C Below 5.7% Simple, Delicious Recipes for Reclaiming Your Health." This section will guide you through the best ways to make the most of this cookbook, ensuring you get the maximum benefit from every recipe and tip included.

Navigating the Cookbook

This cookbook is organized into clearly defined parts, each focusing on a different meal type or dietary need. Here's a quick overview to help you find your way:

Part 1: Getting Started Essential information on stocking your kitchen, cooking tips, and meal planning.

Part 2: Breakfast Delights Energizing and nutritious breakfast options to kick start your day.

Part 3: Energizing Lunches Midday meals that are both satisfying and blood sugar friendly.

Part 4: Satisfying Dinners Delicious dinners that keep you full and help maintain stable blood sugar levels.

Part 5: Snacks and Appetizers Tasty and healthy snacks for between meals.

Part 6: Guilt Free Desserts Sweet treats that you can enjoy without guilt.

Part 7: Smoothies and Beverages Refreshing drinks to complement your meals.

Part 8: Holiday and Special Occasion Meals Festive recipes for special times.

Part 9: Tips and Tricks for Long Term Success Advice on staying motivated and managing diabetes over the long term.

Part 10: Resources and References Additional resources to support your journey.

CHOOSING THE RIGHT RECIPES

Each recipe in this cookbook is designed to help you manage your Type 2 diabetes effectively. When selecting recipes, consider the following:

Nutritional Balance: Look for recipes that offer a good balance of protein, healthy fats, and fiber, while keeping carbs and sugars low.

Personal Preferences: Choose meals that appeal to your taste buds. The more you enjoy the food, the easier it will be to stick to your dietary plan.

Meal Planning: Plan your meals ahead of time using the recipes provided. This will help you stay on track and avoid unhealthy food choices.

Meal Planning and Preparation

Meal planning is a crucial part of managing diabetes. Use the following tips to get started:

Weekly Planning: Set aside time each week to plan your meals. Make a grocery list based on the recipes you want to try.

Batch Cooking: Prepare larger portions of certain dishes and store them in the refrigerator or freezer for easy access throughout the week.

Stay Flexible: Life can be unpredictable. Keep a few quick and easy recipes on hand for days when you're short on time.

Cooking Tips and Techniques

Cooking for diabetes management doesn't have to be complicated. Here are some tips to help you:

Portion Control: Pay attention to portion sizes to avoid overeating. The recipes include recommended serving sizes.

Substitute Smartly: If you have dietary restrictions or preferences, feel free to substitute ingredients. For example, use almond flour instead of regular flour or stevia instead of sugar.

Stay Hydrated: Drinking plenty of water is essential for overall health and can help control blood sugar levels.

Staying Motivated

Adopting a new way of eating can be challenging. Here are some ways to stay motivated:

Track Your Progress: Keep a food diary to track what you eat and how it affects your blood sugar levels.

Set Realistic Goals: Set achievable goals and celebrate your successes, no matter how small.

Find Support: Connect with others who are also managing diabetes. Support groups, online forums, and social media communities can provide encouragement and tips.

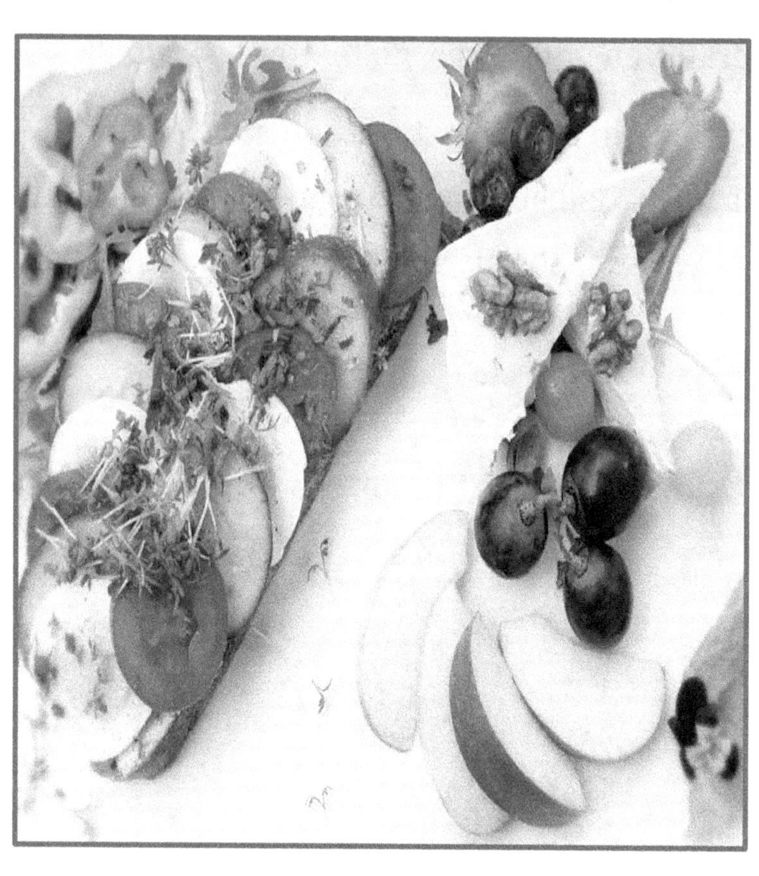

PART 1: GETTING STARTED

Stocking Your Diabetic Friendly Kitchen

Creating a diabetic friendly kitchen is a crucial step towards successfully managing your Type 2 diabetes. By having the right ingredients and tools on hand, you'll make it easier to prepare healthy, delicious meals that support your dietary goals. Here's how to stock your kitchen for success:

Essential Pantry Staples

A well-stocked pantry ensures you're always prepared to make nutritious meals. Keep these staples on hand:

Whole Grains:

- Quinoa
- Brown rice

- Oats

- Barley

- Whole grain pasta

Legumes:

- Lentils

- Chickpeas

- Black beans

- Kidney beans

- Pinto beans

Nuts and Seeds:

- Almonds

- Walnuts

- Chia seeds

- Flaxseeds

- Pumpkin seeds

Healthy Oils and Fats:

- Extra virgin olive oil

- Avocado oil

- Coconut oil

- Nut butters (almond, peanut)

Canned Goods:

- Lowsodium tomatoes

- Tuna or salmon in water

- Coconut milk (unsweetened)

- Vegetable broth (lowsodium)

Flours and Baking Essentials:

- Almond flour

- Coconut flour

- Whole wheat flour

- Baking powder

- Baking soda

Herbs and Spices:

- Cinnamon

- Turmeric

- Cumin
- Paprika
- Basil
- Oregano
- Rosemary

Sweeteners:

- Stevia
- Monk fruit sweetener
- Erythritol

Fresh and Frozen Essentials

Fresh and frozen items are vital for adding variety and nutrition to your meals. Aim to keep the following stocked:

Fresh Produce:

- Leafy greens (spinach, kale, arugula)
- Cruciferous vegetables (broccoli, cauliflower, Brussels sprouts)

- Berries (strawberries, blueberries, raspberries)
- Apples and pears
- Avocados
- Tomatoes
- Cucumbers
- Bell peppers

Frozen Produce:

- Mixed vegetables
- Berries
- Spinach
- Green beans

Proteins:

- Lean meats (chicken breast, turkey)
- Fish (salmon, cod, tilapia)
- Eggs
- Tofu and tempeh
- Low-fat dairy (Greek yogurt, cottage cheese)

Kitchen Tools and Gadgets

Having the right tools can make cooking easier and more enjoyable. Consider adding these to your kitchen:

Cutting Boards and Knives:

- High-quality chef's knife
- Paring knife
- Cutting boards (preferably wooden or plastic)

Cookware:

- Nonstick frying pan
- Cast iron skillet
- Saucepan
- Stockpot

Baking Tools:

- Baking sheets
- Muffin tin

- Loaf pan

Small Appliances:

- Blender
- Food processor
- Slow cooker
- Instant pot or pressure cooker

Measuring Tools:

- Measuring cups
- Measuring spoons
- Kitchen scale

Storage Containers:

- Glass or BPAfree plastic containers
- Mason jars
- Ziptop bags

Tips for Smart Shopping

When shopping for your diabetic friendly kitchen, keep these tips in mind:

1. Read Labels: Look for products with low added sugars, minimal processed ingredients, and low sodium content.

2. Shop the Perimeter: Most fresh, whole foods are located around the perimeter of the store. Focus your shopping here to avoid processed items.

3. Plan Ahead: Make a shopping list based on your meal plan for the week to avoid impulse buys and ensure you have everything you need.

4. Buy in Bulk: Purchase nonperishable items like grains, legumes, and nuts in bulk to save money and reduce the frequency of your shopping trips.

Essential Cooking Tips for Beginners

Embarking on a culinary journey to manage your Type 2 diabetes can be both exciting and overwhelming, especially if you're new to cooking. To help you get started, here are some essential cooking tips that will make preparing healthy, delicious meals a breeze.

Start Simple

When you're new to cooking, it's best to start with simple recipes that require minimal ingredients and steps. As you gain confidence, you can gradually try more complex dishes. Remember, it's better to master a few basic recipes than to struggle with complicated ones.

Read Recipes Thoroughly

Before you begin cooking, read the entire recipe from start to finish. This will help you understand the steps involved, the ingredients needed, and the cooking times. Having a clear picture of the process will make cooking smoother and more enjoyable.

Practice Mise en Place

Mise en place, a French term meaning "everything in its place," involves prepping and organizing all your ingredients before you start cooking. Chop vegetables, measure spices, and gather utensils so everything is ready to go. This practice helps prevent mistakes and makes the cooking process more efficient.

Invest in Quality Tools

Good kitchen tools can make a significant difference in your cooking experience. Invest in a few high-quality items, such as a sharp chef's knife, a cutting board, and a nonstick frying pan. These tools will make preparation easier and more enjoyable.

Master Basic Techniques

Learn a few basic cooking techniques that form the foundation of many recipes:

Chopping and Slicing: Practice safe knife skills to chop and slice vegetables and fruits efficiently.

Sautéing: Use a small amount of oil in a pan over medium heat to cook vegetables and proteins quickly.

Boiling and Simmering: Understand the difference between a rolling boil (high heat) and a gentle simmer (low heat) for cooking grains, pasta, and soups.

Roasting: Use the oven to roast vegetables and meats, which enhances their flavors.

Season Properly

Seasoning is key to making your dishes flavorful and enjoyable. Use herbs, spices, and a small amount of salt to enhance the taste of your food. Experiment with different seasonings to find combinations you love. Fresh herbs and spices can make a big difference in the taste of your meals.

Taste as You Go

As you cook, taste your food periodically to check for seasoning and flavor balance. This allows you to adjust the seasoning as needed and ensures the final dish tastes just right. Remember to use clean utensils for tasting to maintain hygiene.

Embrace Healthy Cooking Methods

Choose cooking methods that retain nutrients and minimize the need for added fats and sugars:

Steaming: Cook vegetables with steam to preserve their nutrients and natural flavors.

Grilling: Grill lean meats and vegetables for a smoky, charred flavor without excess fat.

Baking: Bake proteins and vegetables to achieve a crispy texture without frying.

Stir-frying: Quickly cook thinly sliced ingredients in a small amount of oil over high heat.

Control Portions

Managing portion sizes is crucial for diabetes management. Use measuring cups and a kitchen scale to ensure you're eating appropriate portions. Serve meals on smaller plates to help control portion sizes visually.

Experiment and Have Fun

Cooking should be enjoyable, so don't be afraid to experiment with new ingredients and recipes. Make it a fun and creative activity rather than a chore. Trying new things will keep your meals exciting and prevent boredom.

Stay Organized and Clean

Keep your cooking area clean and organized. Wash dishes and utensils as you go to avoid a large mess at the end. A tidy kitchen makes cooking more pleasant and less stressful.

Learn from Mistakes

Everyone makes mistakes in the kitchen, especially when they're learning. Don't be discouraged by mishaps. Instead, view them as learning opportunities and try to understand what went wrong so you can improve next time.

Meal Planning and Preparation

Effective meal planning and preparation are key to managing Type 2 diabetes while maintaining a balanced and enjoyable diet. By organizing your meals and preparing them in advance, you can make healthier choices, save time, and reduce the stress of daily cooking. Here's a guide to help you plan and prepare your meals efficiently.

Set Up a Meal Planning Routine

Determine Your Goals:

Decide what you want to achieve with your meal plan, such as controlling blood sugar levels, losing weight, or simply eating healthier.

Choose a Planning Frequency:

Plan your meals weekly or biweekly. Weekly planning is often more manageable and allows for more flexibility.

Create a Meal Plan Template:

Use a meal planning template or app to organize your meals. Include breakfast, lunch, dinner, and snacks.

Develop a Balanced Meal Plan

Incorporate a range of protein sources (lean meats, fish, legumes), healthy fats (nuts, avocados), and lowcarb vegetables (leafy greens, cruciferous vegetables).

Plan for Every Meal: Ensure each meal includes a balance of protein, healthy fats, and fiber. Aim for meals that are low in added sugars and refined carbs.

Consider Portion Sizes: Use portion control to manage calorie intake and maintain blood sugar levels. Follow recommended serving sizes and adjust according to your specific needs.

Plan for Leftovers: Cook larger batches of meals to have leftovers for quick and easy meals on busy days.

Make a Grocery List

Check what you already have to avoid buying duplicates. Take note of ingredients that need replenishing.

Create a Shopping List: Write down the ingredients needed for your meal plan. Group items by category (produce, dairy, meats) to streamline your shopping trip.

Stick to Your List: Avoid impulse purchases by sticking to your list. Focus on whole foods and avoid processed items high in sugars and unhealthy fats.

Prep Ingredients in Advance

Wash and Chop Vegetables: Wash and cut vegetables for the week. Store them in airtight containers in the fridge to save time during meal preparation.

Cook in Batches: Prepare larger quantities of staples like grains (quinoa, brown rice) and proteins (chicken, beans). Store them in the refrigerator or freezer for quick meals.

Prepare Snacks: Portion out healthy snacks like nuts, fruits, and yogurt into single servings. Store them in grab and go containers for easy access.

Use Timesaving Techniques

Invest in Kitchen Gadgets: Utilize tools like slow cookers, instant pots, and air fryers to simplify cooking and reduce preparation time.

Embrace One Pan Meals: Prepare meals that require minimal cleanup, such as sheet pan dinners and one pot meals. These are convenient and reduce cooking time.

Prepare Freezer Friendly Meals: Make and freeze meals like soups, stews, and casseroles.

This is a great way to have healthy options readily available.

Stay Flexible and Adjust as Needed

Be Prepared for Changes: Life can be unpredictable. Have a few quick and easy recipes or precooked meals on hand for days when your plans change.

Adjust Based on Feedback: Monitor how different meals affect your blood sugar levels and overall wellbeing. Adjust your meal plan based on what works best for you.

Keep it Enjoyable

Keep your meal plan interesting by incorporating new recipes and ingredients. This can prevent meal fatigue and make cooking more enjoyable.

Involve family members in meal planning and preparation. This can make the process more fun and help everyone stay committed to healthy eating.

Acknowledge and celebrate your progress, whether it's sticking to your meal plan or mastering a new recipe. Positive reinforcement can keep you motivated.

PART 2: BREAKFAST DELIGHTS

Berry Bliss Smoothie Bowl

This Berry Bliss Smoothie Bowl is a refreshing and nutritious way to start your day. Packed with antioxidants from fresh berries and topped with healthy seeds and nuts, it's not only delicious but also helps to keep your blood sugar levels stable.

Perfect for breakfast or a midday snack

Ingredients

Smoothie Base:

- 1 cup unsweetened almond milk (or other low carb milk)
- 1 cup fresh or frozen mixed berries (such as strawberries, blueberries, raspberries)

- 1 small banana (or 1/2 avocado for lower carbs)
- 1 tablespoon chia seeds
- 1 tablespoon almond butter (optional for extra creaminess)

Toppings:

- 1/4 cup granola (sugar free or low sugar)
- 2 tablespoons sliced almonds
- 2 tablespoons fresh berries
- 1 tablespoon shredded coconut (unsweetened)
- A drizzle of honey or a few drops of stevia (optional, for added sweetness)

Instructions

Prepare the Smoothie Base:

- In a blender, combine the unsweetened almond milk, mixed berries, banana (or avocado), chia seeds, and almond butter (if using).

- Blend until smooth and creamy. If the mixture is too thick, you can add a bit more almond milk to reach your desired consistency.

Assemble the Smoothie Bowl: Pour the smoothie base into a bowl, smoothing it out with a spoon.

Add Toppings:

- Sprinkle the granola evenly over the top of the smoothie base.
- Add the sliced almonds, fresh berries, and shredded coconut.
- Drizzle with a small amount of honey or stevia if you prefer additional sweetness.

Serve: Enjoy immediately for the best texture and flavor.

Tips

Berry Variations: Feel free to use any combination of berries you like. Fresh or frozen berries work well.

Low Carb Option: If you're looking to reduce carbs further, use half an avocado instead of the banana for creaminess and extra healthy fats.

Make Ahead: You can prepare the smoothie base ahead of time and store it in the refrigerator for up to 24 hours. Add the toppings just before serving.

Veggie Packed Omelet

This Veggie Packed Omelet is a fantastic way to start your day with a nutritious and satisfying meal. Full of colorful vegetables and packed with protein, it's a perfect breakfast option for managing Type 2 diabetes. This omelet is easy to prepare and can be customized with your favorite veggies.

Ingredients

Omelet:

- 3 large eggs
- 1 tablespoon olive oil or cooking spray
- 1/4 cup diced onion
- 1/4 cup diced bell pepper (any color)
- 1/4 cup diced tomato
- 1/2 cup fresh spinach leaves
- 1/4 cup shredded cheese (optional, use a low-fat cheese if desired)
- Salt and black pepper to taste
- 1/4 teaspoon dried oregano or basil (optional)

Toppings (optional):

- Fresh herbs (parsley, chives, or cilantro)
- Sliced avocado
- A dollop of Greek yogurt

Instructions

Prepare the Vegetables: Dice the onion, bell pepper, and tomato. Wash and pat dry the spinach leaves.

Cook the Vegetables:

- Heat the olive oil in a nonstick skillet over medium heat. Add the diced onion and bell pepper. Cook for about 34 minutes, until softened.
- Add the diced tomato and cook for an additional 2 minutes.

- Stir in the spinach leaves and cook until wilted. Remove the vegetables from the skillet and set aside.

Prepare the Eggs: In a bowl, whisk the eggs until well combined. Season with salt, black pepper, and dried oregano or basil if using.

Cook the Omelet:

- Wipe the skillet clean and add a bit more olive oil or cooking spray. Heat over medium heat.
- Pour the beaten eggs into the skillet, tilting to spread them evenly. Let the eggs cook undisturbed for about 12 minutes, until they begin to set around the edges.

Add the Vegetables:

- Once the edges of the omelet are set but the center is still slightly runny, spread the cooked vegetables evenly over one half of the omelet.

- If using, sprinkle the shredded cheese over the vegetables.

Fold and Finish Cooking: Carefully fold the other half of the omelet over the filling. Cook for an additional 12 minutes, until the eggs are fully set and the cheese (if using) is melted.

Serve: Slide the omelet onto a plate. Garnish with fresh herbs, sliced avocado, or a dollop of Greek yogurt if desired.

Almond Flour Pancakes

These Almond Flour Pancakes are a delicious and low carb alternative to traditional pancakes. Perfect for managing Type 2 diabetes, they're light, fluffy, and packed with protein and healthy fats. Enjoy them for breakfast or as a tasty treat any time of day!

Ingredients

For the Pancakes:

- 1 cup almond flour
- 1/4 cup coconut flour
- 1 tablespoon baking powder
- 1/4 teaspoon salt
- 2 large eggs
- 1/2 cup unsweetened almond milk (or other low carb milk)
- 2 tablespoons melted coconut oil or butter
- 1 teaspoon vanilla extract
- 1 tablespoon maple syrup or a few drops of liquid stevia (optional, for sweetness)

For Cooking: Additional coconut oil or butter for the pan

For Serving (optional):

- Fresh berries

- Sugar free syrup
- Greek yogurt
- A sprinkle of nuts or seeds

Instructions

Mix Dry Ingredients: In a large bowl, whisk together the almond flour, coconut flour, baking powder, and salt.

Combine Wet Ingredients: In another bowl, beat the eggs. Add the unsweetened almond milk, melted coconut oil (or butter), vanilla extract, and maple syrup or liquid stevia if using. Mix well.

Combine Wet and Dry Ingredients: Pour the wet ingredients into the dry ingredients and stir until just combined. The batter will be slightly thick, but should be pourable. If it's too thick, add a bit more almond milk.

Heat the Pan: Heat a nonstick skillet or griddle over medium heat. Add a small amount of coconut oil or butter to the pan, swirling to coat the surface.

Cook the Pancakes: Pour 1/4 cup of batter onto the skillet for each pancake. Cook until bubbles form on the surface and the edges look set, about 23 minutes. Flip and cook for another 12 minutes, until golden brown and cooked through. Repeat with the remaining batter.

Serve: Serve the pancakes warm with your choice of toppings, such as fresh berries, sugarfree syrup, Greek yogurt, or a sprinkle of nuts or seeds.

Tips

- Consistency Adjustment: If the batter is too thick, add a little more almond milk, one tablespoon at a time, until you reach the desired consistency.

- Flavored Pancakes: For a twist, add a pinch of cinnamon or a handful of sugarfree chocolate chips to the batter.
- Make Ahead: Pancakes can be made in advance and stored in the refrigerator for up to 3 days or frozen for up to 3 months. Reheat in a toaster or oven.

Chia Seed Pudding with Fresh Berries

Chia Seed Pudding with Fresh Berries is a delicious and nutritious dessert or breakfast option that's perfect for managing Type 2 diabetes. Packed with fiber, protein, and antioxidants, this pudding is easy to prepare and can be customized with your favorite berries. It's a satisfying treat that helps maintain stable blood sugar levels.

Ingredients

For the Pudding:

- 1/4 cup chia seeds
- 1 cup unsweetened almond milk (or other low carb milk)
- 1 tablespoon maple syrup or a few drops of liquid stevia (optional, for sweetness)
- 1/2 teaspoon vanilla extract

For Topping:

- 1/2 cup fresh berries (such as strawberries, blueberries, raspberries, or blackberries)
- A sprinkle of sliced almonds or nuts (optional)
- A dollop of Greek yogurt (optional)

Instructions

Prepare the Chia Seed Mixture: In a medium bowl, combine the chia seeds, unsweetened almond milk, maple syrup (if using), and vanilla extract. Stir well to mix.

Let it Set: Cover the bowl and refrigerate for at least 2 hours or overnight. The chia seeds will absorb the liquid and swell, creating a pudding like texture. Stir once or twice during the first 30 minutes to prevent clumping.

Serve the Pudding: After the pudding has set, give it a good stir. If it's too thick, you can add a bit more almond milk to reach your desired consistency.

Top with Fresh Berries: Divide the chia seed pudding into serving bowls or glasses. Top with fresh berries and a sprinkle of sliced almonds or nuts if desired. Add a dollop of Greek yogurt for extra creaminess and protein.

Enjoy: Serve immediately or keep it refrigerated until ready to eat. This pudding is best enjoyed cold.

Tips

- Sweetness Adjustment: Adjust the sweetness to your taste. If you prefer a sweeter pudding, add more maple syrup or stevia, but keep in mind that excessive sweeteners can impact blood sugar levels.

- Flavor Variations: Try adding a pinch of cinnamon or nutmeg for extra flavor. You can also mix in a tablespoon of cocoa powder for a chocolate version.

- Berry Choices: Use a mix of your favorite berries for a colorful and flavorful topping. Frozen berries can also be used, but let them thaw slightly before adding.

Greek Yogurt Parfait

This Greek Yogurt Parfait is a delicious and nutritious choice for breakfast or a snack, ideal for managing Type 2 diabetes. Packed with protein from Greek yogurt, fiber from fresh fruit and nuts, and a touch of sweetness, this parfait is both satisfying and blood sugar friendly.

Ingredients

For the Parfait:

- 1 cup plain Greek yogurt (nonfat or low-fat)
- 1/2 cup fresh berries (such as strawberries, blueberries, raspberries, or blackberries)
- 1/4 cup granola (low sugar or sugar free)
- 2 tablespoons sliced almonds or walnuts
- 1 tablespoon chia seeds (optional)
- 1 tablespoon honey or a few drops of liquid stevia (optional, for sweetness)
- 1/2 teaspoon vanilla extract (optional)

Instructions

Prepare the Yogurt: In a bowl, mix the Greek yogurt with honey or liquid stevia if using, and vanilla extract if desired. Stir well to combine.

Layer the Parfait:

- In a serving glass or bowl, start with a layer of Greek yogurt at the bottom.
- Add a layer of fresh berries on top of the yogurt.
- Sprinkle a layer of granola over the berries.
- Add a layer of sliced almonds or walnuts.

Add Optional Chia Seeds: If using chia seeds, sprinkle them on top of the nut layer.

Repeat Layers: Repeat the layers until you reach the top of the glass or bowl, ending with a layer of fresh berries and a sprinkle of granola.

Serve: Enjoy immediately or refrigerate for up to a few hours. The parfait can be made ahead of time, but add the granola just before serving to keep it crunchy.

Tips

Yogurt Choice: Choose plain Greek yogurt to avoid added sugars. If you prefer a bit of sweetness, add honey or stevia to taste.

Berry Variations: Use a mix of berries for added flavor and nutritional benefits. Frozen berries can be used, but let them thaw slightly before adding to the parfait.

Granola Options: Look for granola with low or no added sugar. You can also use nuts or seeds for a crunchy topping if you prefer.

PART 3: ENERGIZING LUNCHES

Grilled Chicken and Quinoa Salad

This Grilled Chicken and Quinoa Salad is a hearty and nutritious meal that's perfect for managing Type 2 diabetes. Packed with lean protein, whole grains, and fresh vegetables, it's a balanced option that's both satisfying and full of flavor. This salad is great for lunch, dinner, or meal prep!

Ingredients

For the Salad:

- 2 boneless, skinless chicken breasts
- 1 tablespoon olive oil
- Salt and black pepper to taste
- 1 teaspoon garlic powder
- 1/2 teaspoon paprika

- 1 cup quinoa

- 2 cups water or low sodium chicken broth

- 1 cup cherry tomatoes, halved

- 1/2 cucumber, diced

- 1/2 red bell pepper, diced

- 1/4 red onion, finely chopped

- 1/4 cup crumbled feta cheese (optional)

- 1/4 cup chopped fresh parsley or cilantro

For the Dressing:

- 3 tablespoons olive oil

- 2 tablespoons lemon juice (about 1 lemon)

- 1 teaspoon Dijon mustard

- 1 teaspoon honey or a few drops of liquid stevia (optional, for sweetness)

- 1 clove garlic, minced

- Salt and black pepper to taste

Instructions

Grill the Chicken:

- Preheat your grill or grill pan to medium high heat.
- Brush the chicken breasts with olive oil and season with salt, black pepper, garlic powder, and paprika.
- Grill the chicken for about 68 minutes per side, or until the internal temperature reaches 165°F (74°C) and the chicken is cooked through.
- Remove the chicken from the grill and let it rest for 5 minutes before slicing.

Cook the Quinoa:

- Rinse the quinoa under cold water.
- In a medium saucepan, bring 2 cups of water or chicken broth to a boil. Add the quinoa, reduce the heat to low, cover, and

simmer for about 15 minutes, or until the quinoa is cooked and the liquid is absorbed.

- Fluff the quinoa with a fork and let it cool slightly.

Prepare the Salad Ingredients: While the quinoa is cooling, prepare the vegetables: halve the cherry tomatoes, dice the cucumber and bell pepper, and finely chop the red onion.

Chop the grilled chicken into bite sized pieces.

Make the Dressing: In a small bowl or jar, whisk together the olive oil, lemon juice, Dijon mustard, honey or liquid stevia (if using), minced garlic, salt, and black pepper until well combined.

Assemble the Salad:

- In a large bowl, combine the cooked quinoa, grilled chicken, cherry tomatoes, cucumber, red bell pepper, red onion, and chopped parsley or cilantro.

- Pour the dressing over the salad and toss gently to combine.
- If using, sprinkle crumbled feta cheese on top.

Serve: Serve the salad immediately or chill in the refrigerator until ready to serve. This salad can be stored in the refrigerator for up to 3 days.

Tips

- Grilled Chicken Alternative: If you prefer, you can also bake or pan sear the chicken.
- Vegetable Variations: Feel free to add or substitute other vegetables such as avocado, spinach, or olives to suit your taste.
- Meal Prep: This salad is great for meal prep. Prepare the quinoa and chicken in advance, and assemble the salad just before eating.

Energizing Lunches

For managing Type 2 diabetes and keeping your energy levels up throughout the day, it's important to choose lunches that are balanced, nutrient dense, and satisfying. Here are some great recipes for energizing lunches that are designed to provide sustained energy and stable blood sugar levels.

Turkey and Avocado Wrap

A low carb, protein rich wrap with healthy fats and fresh vegetables, perfect for a quick and energizing lunch.

Ingredients:

- 1 whole wheat or low carb wrap
- 34 slices of turkey breast
- 1/2 avocado, sliced
- 1/2 cup spinach leaves
- 1/4 cup shredded carrots

- 1 tablespoon hummus or Greek yogurt

Instructions:

1. Spread hummus or Greek yogurt over the wrap.
2. Layer with turkey slices, avocado, spinach, and carrots.
3. Roll up tightly, slice in half, and enjoy!

Mediterranean Chickpea Bowl

This Mediterranean Chickpea Bowl is a delicious, nutrient packed meal that's perfect for lunch or dinner. It's full of fresh vegetables, protein rich chickpeas, and a zesty dressing that ties everything together. Not only is it flavorful and satisfying, but it's also diabetes friendly, helping you maintain stable blood sugar levels while enjoying a delightful dish.

Ingredients:

For the Bowl:

- 1 can (15 oz) chickpeas, drained and rinsed
- 1 cup cooked quinoa
- 1 cup cherry tomatoes, halved
- 1 cucumber, diced
- 1/4 red onion, thinly sliced
- 1/2 cup Kalamata olives, pitted and halved
- 1/4 cup crumbled feta cheese
- 1/4 cup chopped fresh parsley

For the Dressing:

- 3 tablespoons olive oil
- 2 tablespoons lemon juice
- 1 garlic clove, minced
- 1 teaspoon dried oregano
- Salt and black pepper to taste

Instructions:

Prepare the Dressing: In a small bowl, whisk together olive oil, lemon juice, minced garlic, dried oregano, salt, and black pepper. Set aside.

Assemble the Bowl: In a large bowl, combine chickpeas, cooked quinoa, cherry tomatoes, cucumber, red onion, Kalamata olives, feta cheese, and chopped parsley.

Dress the Salad: Pour the dressing over the chickpea and vegetable mixture. Toss gently to ensure everything is well coated with the dressing.

Serve: Divide the Mediterranean Chickpea Bowl into individual serving bowls. Serve immediately, or refrigerate for up to 2 days for a convenient and healthy meal option.

Nutritional Information:

- Serving Size: 1 bowl
- Calories: 350
- Carbohydrates: 45g
- Protein: 12g
- Fat: 14g
- Fiber: 10g
- Sugars: 6g

Tips:

- For added protein, you can include grilled chicken or tofu.
- Adjust the vegetables according to your preferences or seasonal availability.
- The dressing can be made in advance and stored in the refrigerator for up to a week.

Lentil and Vegetable Soup

This Lentil and Vegetable Soup is hearty, nutritious, and perfect for a cozy meal. Packed with fiber rich lentils and a variety of vegetables, it's not only delicious but also great for maintaining stable blood sugar levels. This soup is easy to prepare and makes a wonderful addition to your diabetes friendly recipe collection.

Ingredients:

- 1 tablespoon olive oil
- 1 medium onion, chopped
- 2 garlic cloves, minced
- 2 carrots, diced
- 2 celery stalks, diced
- 1 zucchini, diced
- 1 cup dried green or brown lentils, rinsed and drained
- 1 can (14.5 oz) diced tomatoes, with juices

- 6 cups low sodium vegetable broth
- 1 teaspoon dried thyme
- 1 teaspoon dried oregano
- 1 bay leaf
- Salt and black pepper to taste
- 2 cups fresh spinach or kale, chopped
- Juice of 1 lemon
- Fresh parsley, chopped (for garnish)

Instructions:

Sauté the Vegetables: In a large pot, heat the olive oil over medium heat. Add the chopped onion and cook until translucent, about 5 minutes. Add the minced garlic and cook for another minute.

Add the Vegetables and Lentils: Stir in the diced carrots, celery, and zucchini. Cook for about 5 minutes, stirring occasionally. Add the rinsed lentils and can of diced tomatoes (with juices).

Simmer the Soup: Pour in the vegetable broth and add the dried thyme, dried oregano, bay leaf, salt, and black pepper. Bring the soup to a boil, then reduce the heat to low and let it simmer, covered, for about 30 minutes or until the lentils and vegetables are tender.

Add Greens and Lemon Juice: Stir in the chopped spinach or kale and let it cook for another 5 minutes until the greens are wilted. Remove the bay leaf and stir in the lemon juice.

Serve: Ladle the soup into bowls and garnish with fresh parsley. Serve hot.

Nutritional Information:

- Serving Size: 1 bowl (approximately 1.5 cups)
- Calories: 200
- Carbohydrates: 32g
- Protein: 10g

- Fat: 4g
- Fiber: 12g
- Sugars: 7g

Tips:

- This soup can be stored in the refrigerator for up to 5 days or frozen for up to 3 months.
- Feel free to add other vegetables you enjoy, such as bell peppers or green beans.
- For a heartier meal, serve with a side of wholegrain bread.

Stuffed Bell Peppers

Stuffed Bell Peppers are a colorful, nutritious, and satisfying dish perfect for lunch or dinner. This recipe is loaded with lean protein, fiber, and essential nutrients, making it an excellent choice for managing Type 2 diabetes while enjoying a delicious meal.

Ingredients:

- 4 large bell peppers (any color), tops cut off and seeds removed
- 1 tablespoon olive oil
- 1 medium onion, chopped
- 2 garlic cloves, minced
- 1 pound ground turkey or lean ground beef
- 1 cup cooked quinoa or brown rice
- 1 can (14.5 oz) diced tomatoes, with juices
- 1 teaspoon dried oregano
- 1 teaspoon dried basil
- 1 teaspoon smoked paprika
- Salt and black pepper to taste
- 1 cup shredded mozzarella or cheddar cheese (optional)
- Fresh parsley, chopped (for garnish)

Instructions:

Preheat the Oven: Preheat your oven to 375°F (190°C).

Prepare the Bell Peppers: Cut the tops off the bell peppers and remove the seeds and membranes. If needed, slice a small piece off the bottom so they stand upright. Place them in a baking dish.

Cook the Filling:

- In a large skillet, heat the olive oil over medium heat. Add the chopped onion and cook until softened, about 5 minutes. Add the minced garlic and cook for another minute.
- Add the ground turkey or lean ground beef to the skillet. Cook until browned and fully cooked, breaking it up with a spoon as it cooks.
- Stir in the cooked quinoa or brown rice, diced tomatoes (with juices), dried oregano, dried

basil, smoked paprika, salt, and black pepper. Cook for another 5 minutes, allowing the flavors to meld.

Stuff the Peppers: Spoon the filling mixture into each bell pepper, packing it in tightly. If using, sprinkle shredded cheese on top of each stuffed pepper.

Bake the Peppers: Cover the baking dish with foil and bake for 30 minutes. Remove the foil and bake for an additional 1015 minutes, or until the peppers are tender and the cheese (if using) is melted and bubbly.

Serve: Garnish the stuffed bell peppers with fresh chopped parsley. Serve hot.

Nutritional Information:

- Serving Size: 1 stuffed pepper
- Calories: 300

- Carbohydrates: 20g

- Protein: 25g

- Fat: 12g

- Fiber: 5g

- Sugars: 6g

Tips:

Feel free to customize the filling with other vegetables such as chopped spinach, zucchini, or mushrooms.

These stuffed bell peppers can be made ahead of time and reheated for a quick and healthy meal.

For a vegetarian option, replace the meat with additional vegetables or plant based protein such as lentils or beans.

PART 4: SATISFYING DINNERS

A Well-balanced dinner is essential for maintaining stable blood sugar levels and ensuring you feel full and satisfied. Here are some delicious and satisfying dinner recipes designed to provide the right mix of nutrients and flavor, perfect for managing Type 2 diabetes.

Baked Salmon with Roasted Vegetables

Baked Salmon with Roasted Vegetables is a simple, nutritious, and delicious meal that's perfect for any day of the week. This dish is rich in omega3 fatty acids, fiber, and essential vitamins, making it an excellent choice for managing Type 2 diabetes while enjoying a flavorful dinner.

Ingredients:

For the Salmon:

- 4 salmon fillets (about 6 oz each)
- 2 tablespoons olive oil
- 2 tablespoons lemon juice
- 2 garlic cloves, minced
- 1 teaspoon dried dill or fresh dill
- Salt and black pepper to taste
- Lemon slices (for garnish)
- Fresh dill (for garnish)

For the Roasted Vegetables:

- 1 large red bell pepper, cut into strips
- 1 large yellow bell pepper, cut into strips
- 1 medium zucchini, sliced
- 1 medium yellow squash, sliced
- 1 red onion, cut into wedges
- 2 cups broccoli florets
- 2 tablespoons olive oil
- 1 teaspoon dried thyme

- 1 teaspoon dried rosemary

- Salt and black pepper to taste

Instructions:

Preheat the Oven: Preheat your oven to 400°F (200°C).

Prepare the Marinade for the Salmon: In a small bowl, whisk together the olive oil, lemon juice, minced garlic, dried dill, salt, and black pepper.

Marinate the Salmon: Place the salmon fillets on a baking sheet lined with parchment paper. Brush the marinade over the salmon fillets, making sure they are well coated. Set aside to marinate while you prepare the vegetables.

Prepare the Vegetables: In a large bowl, combine the red and yellow bell peppers, zucchini, yellow squash, red onion, and broccoli florets. Drizzle with olive oil and sprinkle with dried thyme, dried rosemary, salt, and black pepper. Toss to coat the vegetables evenly.

Arrange the Vegetables and Salmon: Spread the vegetables out in a single layer on a separate baking sheet. Place both baking sheets (with the salmon and vegetables) in the preheated oven.

Bake the vegetables for 2025 minutes or until they are tender and slightly caramelized, stirring once halfway through.

Bake the salmon for 1215 minutes, or until it flakes easily with a fork and is cooked through.

Serve: Remove the salmon and vegetables from the oven. Garnish the salmon with lemon slices and fresh dill. Serve the salmon fillets alongside the roasted vegetables.

Nutritional Information:

- Serving Size: 1 salmon fillet with a portion of vegetables
- Calories: 400
- Carbohydrates: 15g
- Protein: 30g
- Fat: 25g
- Fiber: 6g
- Sugars: 7g

Tips:

Feel free to customize the vegetables according to your preferences or seasonal availability.

For extra flavor, add a splash of balsamic vinegar to the vegetables before roasting.

This dish pairs well with a simple green salad or wholegrain side dish for a complete meal.

Stuffed Zucchini Boats

Stuffed Zucchini Boats are a delightful and healthy way to enjoy a variety of flavors and nutrients in one dish. This recipe is packed with lean protein, fiber, and essential vitamins, making it a fantastic choice for managing Type 2 diabetes while indulging in a delicious meal.

Ingredients:

- 4 medium zucchinis
- 1 tablespoon olive oil
- 1 medium onion, chopped
- 2 garlic cloves, minced
- 1 pound ground turkey or lean ground beef
- 1 cup diced tomatoes (fresh or canned)
- 1/2 cup cooked quinoa or brown rice
- 1 teaspoon dried oregano
- 1 teaspoon dried basil
- 1/2 teaspoon smoked paprika

- Salt and black pepper to taste
- 1/2 cup shredded mozzarella or cheddar cheese (optional)
- Fresh parsley, chopped (for garnish)

Instructions:

Preheat your oven to 375°F (190°C).

Prepare the Zucchinis: Wash the zucchinis and cut them in half lengthwise. Use a spoon to scoop out the center flesh, creating a boat like shape. Set the scooped flesh aside.

Cook the Filling:

- In a large skillet, heat the olive oil over medium heat. Add the chopped onion and cook until softened, about 5 minutes. Add the minced garlic and cook for another minute.

- Add the ground turkey or lean ground beef to the skillet. Cook until browned and fully cooked, breaking it up with a spoon as it cooks.

- Chop the reserved zucchini flesh and add it to the skillet along with the diced tomatoes, cooked quinoa or brown rice, dried oregano, dried basil, smoked paprika, salt, and black pepper. Cook for an additional 5 minutes, allowing the flavors to meld.

Stuff the Zucchini Boats: Place the zucchini boats in a baking dish. Spoon the filling mixture into each zucchini boat, packing it in tightly. If using, sprinkle shredded cheese on top of each stuffed zucchini.

Bake: Cover the baking dish with foil and bake for 2530 minutes. Remove the foil and bake for an additional 1015 minutes, or until the zucchinis are tender and the cheese (if using) is melted and bubbly.

Serve: Garnish the stuffed zucchini boats with fresh chopped parsley. Serve hot.

Nutritional Information:

- Serving Size: 1 stuffed zucchini boat
- Calories: 220
- Carbohydrates: 12g
- Protein: 20g
- Fat: 10g
- Fiber: 4g
- Sugars: 6g

Tips:

Customize the filling with other vegetables such as bell peppers, spinach, or mushrooms.

These stuffed zucchini boats can be made ahead of time and reheated for a quick and healthy meal.

For a vegetarian option, replace the meat with additional vegetables or plantbased protein such as lentils or beans.

Chicken StirFry with Broccoli and Bell Peppers

Chicken StirFry with Broccoli and Bell Peppers is a quick, healthy, and delicious meal perfect for busy weeknights. This recipe is packed with lean protein, colorful vegetables, and a savory sauce, making it an excellent choice for managing Type 2 diabetes while enjoying a flavorful dinner.

Ingredients:

For the Stir-fry:

- 1 tablespoon olive oil or sesame oil
- 1 pound boneless, skinless chicken breasts, cut into thin strips
- 2 cups broccoli florets
- 1 red bell pepper, thinly sliced

- 1 yellow bell pepper, thinly sliced
- 1 medium carrot, julienned
- 3 green onions, sliced
- 2 garlic cloves, minced
- 1 teaspoon fresh ginger, grated

For the Sauce:

- 1/4 cup low sodium soy sauce or tamari
- 2 tablespoons hoisin sauce
- 1 tablespoon rice vinegar
- 1 tablespoon honey or a sugar substitute suitable for cooking
- 1 teaspoon cornstarch (optional, for thickening)
- 1/4 cup water

Instructions:

Prepare the Sauce: In a small bowl, whisk together the soy sauce, hoisin sauce, rice vinegar, honey, cornstarch (if using), and water. Set aside.

Cook the Chicken: Heat the olive oil or sesame oil in a large skillet or wok over medium high heat. Add the chicken strips and cook until browned and cooked through, about 57 minutes. Remove the chicken from the skillet and set aside.

Cook the Vegetables: In the same skillet, add the broccoli florets, red and yellow bell peppers, and carrots. Stir-fry for about 5 minutes until the vegetables are tender crisp. Add the green onions, minced garlic, and grated ginger, and stir-fry for an additional 12 minutes until fragrant.

Combine Chicken and Vegetables:

Return the cooked chicken to the skillet with the vegetables. Pour the sauce over the chicken and vegetables, stirring to coat everything evenly. Cook for another 23 minutes until the sauce thickens and everything is heated through.

Serve: Serve the chicken stir-fry over cooked brown rice, quinoa, or cauliflower rice for a low carb option. Garnish with additional sliced green onions or sesame seeds if desired.

Nutritional Information:

- Serving Size: 1 cup (without rice or additional sides)
- Calories: 250
- Carbohydrates: 12g
- Protein: 30g
- Fat: 10g
- Fiber: 4g
- Sugars: 6g

Tips:

Customize the vegetables according to your preferences or what you have on hand.

For a spicier dish, add a pinch of red pepper flakes or a drizzle of sriracha to the sauce.

This stir-fry can be made ahead and reheated for a quick and healthy meal throughout the week.

Beef and Vegetable Skillet

Beef and Vegetable Skillet is a hearty and nutritious meal that's perfect for busy weeknights. This recipe is packed with lean protein, fiber, and a variety of colorful vegetables, making it a great choice for managing Type 2 diabetes while enjoying a delicious and satisfying dinner.

Ingredients:

- 1 tablespoon olive oil
- 1 pound lean ground beef (90% lean or higher)
- 1 medium onion, chopped

- 2 garlic cloves, minced
- 1 red bell pepper, chopped
- 1 green bell pepper, chopped
- 2 cups broccoli florets
- 1 medium zucchini, sliced
- 1 cup cherry tomatoes, halved
- 1 teaspoon dried oregano
- 1 teaspoon dried basil
- 1/2 teaspoon smoked paprika
- Salt and black pepper to taste
- 1/4 cup grated Parmesan cheese (optional)
- Fresh parsley, chopped (for garnish)

Instructions:

Cook the Beef: Heat the olive oil in a large skillet over medium high heat. Add the ground beef and cook until browned, breaking it up with a spoon as it cooks. Remove the beef from the skillet and set aside, leaving a little bit of fat in the skillet.

Sauté the Aromatics: In the same skillet, add the chopped onion and cook until softened, about 5 minutes. Add the minced garlic and cook for another minute until fragrant.

Cook the Vegetables: Add the red and green bell peppers, broccoli florets, zucchini, and cherry tomatoes to the skillet. Cook for about 810 minutes, stirring occasionally, until the vegetables are tender crisp.

Season and Combine: Return the cooked ground beef to the skillet. Add the dried oregano, dried basil, smoked paprika, salt, and black pepper. Stir well to combine and cook for an additional 23 minutes until everything is heated through.

Serve: If using, sprinkle the grated Parmesan cheese over the top of the skillet. Garnish with fresh chopped parsley. Serve hot.

Nutritional Information:

- Serving Size: 1 cup
- Calories: 280
- Carbohydrates: 10g
- Protein: 25g
- Fat: 15g
- Fiber: 4g
- Sugars: 5g

Tips:

Feel free to customize the vegetables according to your preferences or seasonal availability.

For a spicier version, add a pinch of red pepper flakes or a splash of hot sauce.

This dish can be served over whole grain pasta, quinoa, or cauliflower rice for a more substantial meal.

5. Spaghetti Squash with Turkey Marinara

Spaghetti Squash with Turkey Marinara is a delicious and nutritious alternative to traditional pasta dishes. This recipe combines the mild, slightly sweet flavor of spaghetti squash with a lean turkey marinara sauce, offering a lowercarb option that is perfect for managing Type 2 diabetes.

Ingredients:

For the Spaghetti Squash:

- 1 medium spaghetti squash
- 1 tablespoon olive oil
- Salt and black pepper to taste

For the Turkey Marinara Sauce:

- 1 tablespoon olive oil
- 1 pound lean ground turkey
- 1 medium onion, chopped
- 2 garlic cloves, minced
- 1 can (14.5 oz) diced tomatoes, with juices
- 1 can (6 oz) tomato paste
- 1/2 cup low sodium chicken or vegetable broth
- 1 teaspoon dried oregano
- 1 teaspoon dried basil
- 1/2 teaspoon dried thyme
- 1/2 teaspoon red pepper flakes (optional)
- Salt and black pepper to taste
- 1/4 cup chopped fresh basil or parsley (for garnish)

Instructions:

Prepare the Spaghetti Squash: Preheat your oven to 400°F (200°C).

- Cut the spaghetti squash in half lengthwise and scoop out the seeds. Drizzle the cut sides with olive oil and season with salt and black pepper.
- Place the squash cut side down on a baking sheet lined with parchment paper. Roast in the preheated oven for 4045 minutes, or until the flesh is tender and can be easily shredded with a fork.
- Remove from the oven and let cool slightly. Use a fork to scrape the flesh into spaghetti like strands.

Prepare the Turkey Marinara Sauce:

- While the squash is roasting, heat olive oil in a large skillet over medium heat. Add the chopped onion and cook until softened, about 5 minutes. Add the minced garlic and cook for an additional minute.

- Add the ground turkey to the skillet and cook until browned and fully cooked, breaking it up with a spoon as it cooks.
- Stir in the diced tomatoes, tomato paste, and chicken or vegetable broth. Add the dried oregano, dried basil, dried thyme, red pepper flakes (if using), salt, and black pepper. Simmer the sauce for about 1520 minutes, allowing the flavors to meld and the sauce to thicken.

Serve: Divide the spaghetti squash strands among serving plates. Top with the turkey marinara sauce.

Garnish with chopped fresh basil or parsley.

Nutritional Information:

- Serving Size: 1 cup of spaghetti squash with 1/2 cup of turkey marinara sauce
- Calories: 250
- Carbohydrates: 20g
- Protein: 22g
- Fat: 10g
- Fiber: 6g
- Sugars: 7g

Tips:

For added flavor, sprinkle a bit of grated Parmesan cheese over the top before serving.

You can add vegetables like bell peppers or mushrooms to the marinara sauce for extra nutrients and flavor.

The marinara sauce can be made ahead of time and stored in the refrigerator for up to 4 days or frozen for up to 3 months.

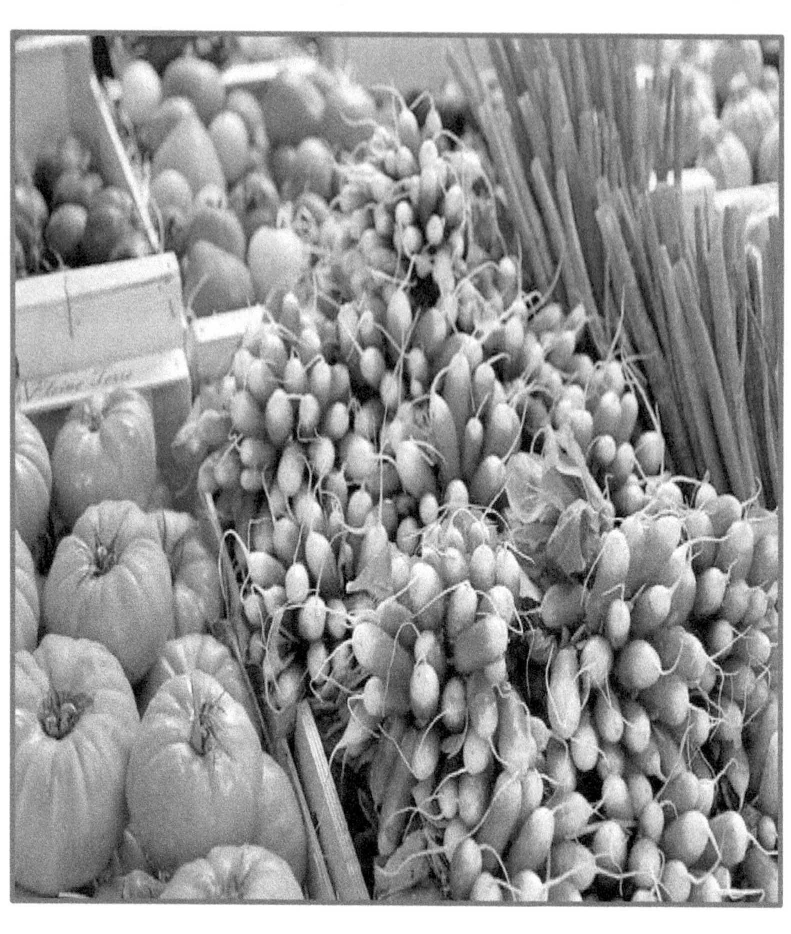

PART 5: SNACKS AND APPETIZERS

For managing Type 2 diabetes, choosing the right snacks and appetizers can help keep blood sugar levels stable and provide sustained energy. Here are some delicious, low carb, and nutritious options perfect for any time of day:

Greek Yogurt and Veggie Dip

A creamy and satisfying dip that pairs perfectly with fresh veggies, making for a nutritious snack.

Ingredients:

- 1 cup plain Greek yogurt (nonfat or lowfat)
- 1 tablespoon olive oil
- 1 tablespoon lemon juice
- 1 teaspoon dried dill or chopped fresh dill
- 1 clove garlic, minced

- Salt and black pepper to taste

For Serving:

- Sliced cucumbers
- Cherry tomatoes
- Carrot sticks
- Bell pepper strips

Instructions:

1. In a bowl, mix Greek yogurt, olive oil, lemon juice, dill, garlic, salt, and pepper.
2. Chill the dip in the refrigerator for at least 30 minutes to allow flavors to meld.
3. Serve with sliced vegetables.

Stuffed Mini Peppers Sweet mini peppers stuffed with a savory mixture of cheese and herbs, perfect for a quick and flavorful bite.

Ingredients:

- 12 mini sweet peppers, halved and seeds removed
- 1/2 cup cream cheese, softened
- 1/4 cup shredded cheddar cheese
- 1 tablespoon chopped fresh parsley
- 1/4 teaspoon garlic powder
- Salt and black pepper to taste

Instructions:

1. Preheat oven to 375°F (190°C).
2. In a bowl, mix cream cheese, cheddar cheese, parsley, garlic powder, salt, and pepper.
3. Fill each mini pepper half with the cheese mixture.
4. Arrange stuffed peppers on a baking sheet and bake for 1520 minutes, until peppers are tender and cheese is melted.

Avocado and Tuna Salad Bites

Delicious and filling, these bites combine creamy avocado with protein packed tuna for a healthy snack or appetizer.

Ingredients:

- 1 can (5 oz) tuna, drained
- 1 ripe avocado, peeled and diced
- 1 tablespoon lemon juice
- 1 tablespoon chopped fresh cilantro or parsley
- Salt and black pepper to taste

For Serving: Sliced cucumber rounds or endive leaves

Instructions:

1. In a bowl, mix tuna, avocado, lemon juice, cilantro, salt, and pepper.

2. Spoon the mixture onto cucumber rounds or endive leaves.

3. Serve immediately.

Roasted Chickpeas Crunchy and flavorful, roasted chickpeas make a great low carb snack with a satisfying crunch.

Ingredients:

- 1 can (15 oz) chickpeas, drained and rinsed
- 1 tablespoon olive oil
- 1 teaspoon smoked paprika
- 1/2 teaspoon garlic powder
- 1/2 teaspoon cumin
- Salt to taste

Instructions:

1. Preheat oven to 400°F (200°C).
2. Pat chickpeas dry with a paper towel.

3. Toss chickpeas with olive oil, paprika, garlic powder, cumin, and salt.

4. Spread on a baking sheet and roast for 2530 minutes, shaking the pan halfway through, until chickpeas are crispy.

Egg Muffins

These versatile egg muffins are packed with protein and vegetables, perfect for a quick and easy snack or appetizer.

Ingredients:

- 6 large eggs
- 1/4 cup milk (unsweetened almond or other low carb milk)
- 1/2 cup diced bell peppers
- 1/2 cup chopped spinach
- 1/4 cup shredded cheese (cheddar, feta, or your choice)
- Salt and black pepper to taste

Instructions:

1. Preheat oven to 375°F (190°C) and grease a muffin tin or line with paper liners.
2. In a bowl, whisk together eggs, milk, salt, and pepper.
3. Divide bell peppers, spinach, and cheese among the muffin tin cups.
4. Pour the egg mixture over the vegetables and cheese.
5. Bake for 2025 minutes, until muffins are set and golden brown.

Cucumber and Hummus Bites

Fresh cucumber slices topped with a dollop of creamy hummus, making for a refreshing and satisfying snack.

Ingredients:

- 1 cucumber, sliced into rounds

- 1/2 cup hummus (store bought or homemade)
- Paprika or fresh herbs for garnish (optional)

Instructions:

1. Spread a small amount of hummus on each cucumber slice.
2. Garnish with paprika or fresh herbs if desired.
3. Serve immediately.

PART 6: GUILT FREE DESSERTS

Indulge in this delicious guilt free desserts that are both satisfying and suitable for managing Type 2 diabetes. Each recipe is designed to be lower in sugar and carbohydrates while still offering a sweet treat to end your meal on a high note.

Berry Chia Seed Jam

Berry Chia Seed Jam is a healthy and delicious alternative to traditional fruit preserves. Using chia seeds as a thickening agent, this jam is naturally sweetened and packed with fiber, antioxidants, and omega 3 fatty acids, making it a great choice for managing Type 2 diabetes.

Ingredients:

- 2 cups fresh or frozen berries (such as strawberries, blueberries, raspberries, or a mix)
- 2 tablespoons maple syrup or honey (or a sugar substitute suitable for cooking)
- 1 tablespoon lemon juice
- 2 tablespoons chia seeds
- 1/2 teaspoon vanilla extract (optional)

Instructions:

Cook the Berries: In a medium saucepan, combine the berries, maple syrup or honey, and lemon juice. Cook over medium heat, stirring occasionally, until the berries have softened and released their juices, about 5 7 minutes.

Mash the Berries: Use a fork or potato masher to mash the berries to your desired consistency.

For a smoother jam, you can use an immersion blender or regular blender to blend the mixture.

Add Chia Seeds: Stir in the chia seeds and continue to cook the mixture for an additional 5 minutes, stirring frequently. The chia seeds will absorb the liquid and help thicken the jam.

Cool and Set: Remove the saucepan from the heat and stir in the vanilla extract, if using. Let the jam cool to room temperature. As it cools, it will continue to thicken.

Store: Transfer the jam to a clean jar or container. Store in the refrigerator for up to 2 weeks. For longer storage, you can freeze the jam for up to 3 months.

Nutritional Information (per 2 tablespoon serving):

- Calories: 50

- Carbohydrates: 12g
- Protein: 1g
- Fat: 1g
- Fiber: 3g
- Sugars: 8g

Tips:

Feel free to use any combination of berries according to your preference or what you have on hand.

Adjust the sweetness to your taste by varying the amount of maple syrup or honey.

For a seed free jam, you can strain out the chia seeds after cooking, though this will reduce the jam's thickening properties and nutritional benefits.

Avocado Chocolate Mousse

Avocado Chocolate Mousse is a rich and creamy dessert that's both indulgent and healthy. Made with ripe avocados, this mousse is naturally sweetened and provides healthy fats, making it a fantastic option for managing Type 2 diabetes while satisfying your sweet tooth.

Ingredients:

- 2 ripe avocados, peeled and pitted
- 1/4 cup unsweetened cocoa powder
- 1/4 cup maple syrup or honey (or a sugar substitute suitable for cooking)
- 1/4 cup almond milk or other unsweetened milk of choice
- 1 teaspoon vanilla extract
- Pinch of salt
- Fresh berries or mint leaves (for garnish, optional)

Instructions:

Blend Ingredients:

In a food processor or blender, combine the avocados, cocoa powder, maple syrup or honey, almond milk, vanilla extract, and a pinch of salt. Blend until smooth and creamy, scraping down the sides as needed.

Adjust Sweetness and Texture:

- Taste the mousse and adjust the sweetness or cocoa powder according to your preference. If the mousse is too thick, add a little more almond milk to achieve your desired consistency.

- Transfer the mousse to serving dishes or bowls. Refrigerate for at least 30 minutes to allow the flavors to meld and the mousse to firm up.

- Garnish with fresh berries or mint leaves, if desired. Serve chilled.

Nutritional Information (per ½ cup serving):

- Calories: 180
- Carbohydrates: 14g
- Protein: 3g
- Fat: 12g
- Fiber: 6g
- Sugars: 7g

Tips:

For a richer chocolate flavor, you can add a bit more cocoa powder.

Experiment with different sweeteners or flavorings, such as a touch of cinnamon or a splash of espresso, for a unique twist.

This mousse can be stored in the refrigerator for up to 3 days, making it a great make ahead dessert.

Baked Apple Slices with Cinnamon

Simple and satisfying baked apple slices with a touch of cinnamon, perfect for a cozy dessert.

Ingredients:

- 2 large apples, cored and sliced thinly
- 1 tablespoon olive oil
- 1 teaspoon ground cinnamon
- 1 tablespoon chopped nuts (optional)

Instructions:

1. Preheat oven to 350°F (175°C).
2. Toss apple slices with olive oil and ground cinnamon. Arrange them in a single layer on a baking sheet.
3. Bake for 15 20 minutes, or until the apples are tender and slightly caramelized.
4. Sprinkle with chopped nuts if desired. Serve warm or at room temperature.

Greek Yogurt with Nuts and Seeds

A quick and easy dessert that's both satisfying and packed with protein and healthy fats.

Ingredients:

- 1 cup plain Greek yogurt
- 2 tablespoons mixed nuts (such as almonds, walnuts, or pecans), chopped
- 1 tablespoon chia seeds
- 1 tablespoon unsweetened shredded coconut (optional)
- A few fresh berries or a drizzle of honey (optional)

Instructions:

1. Scoop Greek yogurt into a bowl.
2. Top with mixed nuts, chia seeds, shredded coconut, and fresh berries or a drizzle of honey if using.

3. Enjoy immediately, or chill in the refrigerator for a refreshing treat.

Coconut Flour Muffins

These low carb, high fiber muffins are perfect for a quick dessert or a sweet snack.

Ingredients:

- 1/2 cup coconut flour
- 1/4 cup almond flour
- 1/2 teaspoon baking powder
- 1/4 teaspoon salt
- 3 large eggs
- 1/4 cup coconut oil, melted
- 1/4 cup unsweetened applesauce
- 1/4 cup honey or a few drops of liquid stevia (optional, for sweetness)
- 1/2 teaspoon vanilla extract

Instructions:

1. Preheat oven to 350°F (175°C) and line a muffin tin with paper liners.
2. In a bowl, whisk together coconut flour, almond flour, baking powder, and salt.
3. In another bowl, mix eggs, melted coconut oil, applesauce, honey or stevia, and vanilla extract.
4. Combine wet and dry ingredients and stir until well mixed.
5. Divide the batter evenly among the muffin cups.
6. Bake for 20 25 minutes, or until a toothpick inserted in the center comes out clean. Allow to cool before serving.

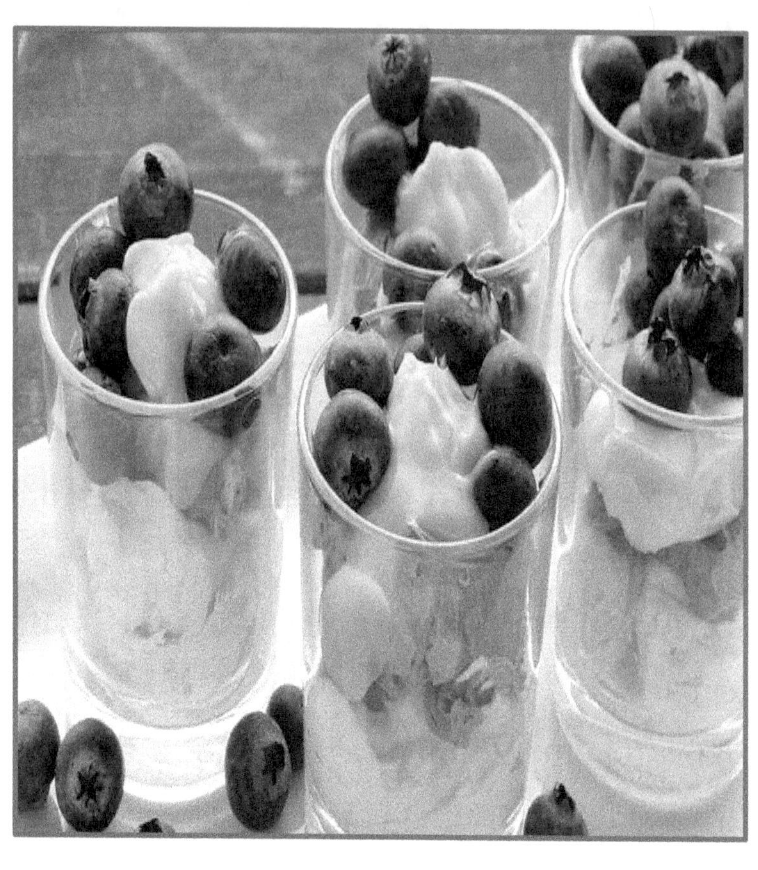

PART 7: SMOOTHIES AND BEVERAGES

Healthy smoothies and beverages can be a great addition to your diet, providing essential nutrients while helping to manage blood sugar levels.

Berry Spinach Smoothie

A nutrient packed smoothie combining berries, spinach, and a hint of yogurt for a refreshing drink that's rich in antioxidants and fiber.

Ingredients:

- 1 cup fresh spinach leaves
- 1/2 cup frozen mixed berries (such as strawberries, blueberries, raspberries)
- 1/2 cup plain Greek yogurt
- 1/2 cup unsweetened almond milk (or other low carb milk)

- 1 tablespoon chia seeds (optional)
- 1/2 teaspoon honey or a few drops of liquid stevia (optional, for sweetness)
- Ice cubes (optional)

Instructions:

1. In a blender, combine spinach, mixed berries, Greek yogurt, almond milk, chia seeds, and honey or stevia if using.
2. Blend until smooth. Add ice cubes if desired and blend again until frothy.
3. Pour into a glass and serve immediately.

Green Detox Smoothie

A light and detoxifying smoothie featuring cucumber, green apple, and a splash of lemon, perfect for a refreshing start to your day.

Ingredients:

- 1/2 cucumber, peeled and sliced

- 1 green apple, cored and sliced
- 1/2 cup kale or spinach
- 1/2 cup unsweetened coconut water
- Juice of 1/2 lemon
- 1 tablespoon fresh ginger, grated
- Ice cubes (optional)

Instructions:

1. Combine cucumber, green apple, kale or spinach, coconut water, lemon juice, and ginger in a blender.
2. Blend until smooth. Add ice cubes if desired and blend again until well combined.
3. Pour into a glass and enjoy!

Creamy Avocado Smoothie

A rich and creamy smoothie that combines avocado with a touch of vanilla and unsweetened almond milk for a satisfying treat.

Ingredients:

- 1/2 ripe avocado
- 1/2 cup plain Greek yogurt
- 1/2 cup unsweetened almond milk
- 1/2 teaspoon vanilla extract
- A few drops of liquid stevia or 1 teaspoon honey (optional, for sweetness)
- Ice cubes (optional)

Instructions:

1. Scoop the avocado into a blender. Add Greek yogurt, almond milk, vanilla extract, and sweetener if using.
2. Blend until smooth and creamy. Add ice cubes if desired and blend again.
3. Serve immediately in a glass.

Cucumber Mint Infused Water

A refreshing and hydrating beverage that's perfect for staying hydrated with a subtle hint of cucumber and mint.

Ingredients:

- 1/2 cucumber, sliced
- A handful of fresh mint leaves
- 1 lemon, sliced
- 4 cups water
- Ice cubes

Instructions:

1. In a pitcher, combine cucumber slices, mint leaves, and lemon slices.
2. Add water and ice cubes.
3. Let the mixture infuse in the refrigerator for at least 1 hour before serving.
4. **Almond Milk Iced Coffee**

A low carb alternative to traditional iced coffee, made with almond milk for a creamy, guilt free treat.

Ingredients:

- 1 cup brewed coffee, cooled
- 1/2 cup unsweetened almond milk
- 1/2 teaspoon vanilla extract
- A few drops of liquid stevia or 1 teaspoon honey (optional, for sweetness)
- Ice cubes

Instructions:

1. In a glass, combine brewed coffee, almond milk, vanilla extract, and sweetener if using.
2. Stir well and add ice cubes.
3. Serve immediately.

Low Sugar Chocolate Smoothie

This Low Sugar Chocolate Smoothie is a creamy and satisfying treat that's perfect for those looking to enjoy a chocolate flavored drink without the added sugars. Packed with nutrients and made with wholesome ingredients, it's a great option for managing Type 2 diabetes while indulging in a delicious beverage.

Ingredients:

- 1 cup unsweetened almond milk or other unsweetened milk of choice
- 1/2 cup plain Greek yogurt (full fat or low fat)
- 1 tablespoon unsweetened cocoa powder
- 1 tablespoon chia seeds
- 1/2 avocado, peeled and pitted
- 1 tablespoon sugar free chocolate syrup or 1 2 teaspoons of a sugar substitute (optional)

- 1/2 teaspoon vanilla extract
- A handful of ice cubes

Instructions:

1. Combine Ingredients: In a blender, combine the almond milk, Greek yogurt, cocoa powder, chia seeds, avocado, sugar free chocolate syrup (if using), and vanilla extract.

2. **Blend:** Blend until smooth and creamy, making sure the avocado and chia seeds are well incorporated. Add ice cubes and blend again until the smoothie reaches your desired consistency.

3. Adjust Sweetness: Taste the smoothie and adjust the sweetness if needed. You can add a bit more sugar substitute or syrup if you prefer a sweeter taste.

4. **Serve:** Pour the smoothie into a glass and enjoy immediately.

Nutritional Information (per 1 serving):

- Calories: 220
- Carbohydrates: 16g
- Protein: 10g
- Fat: 14g
- Fiber: 7g
- Sugars: 5g

Tips:

For added nutrition, you can toss in a handful of spinach or kale. The flavor will be masked by the chocolate, and you'll get extra vitamins and minerals.

To make the smoothie thicker, freeze the avocado before using or add a few more ice cubes.

You can use different milk alternatives like soy or oat milk based on your preference and dietary needs.

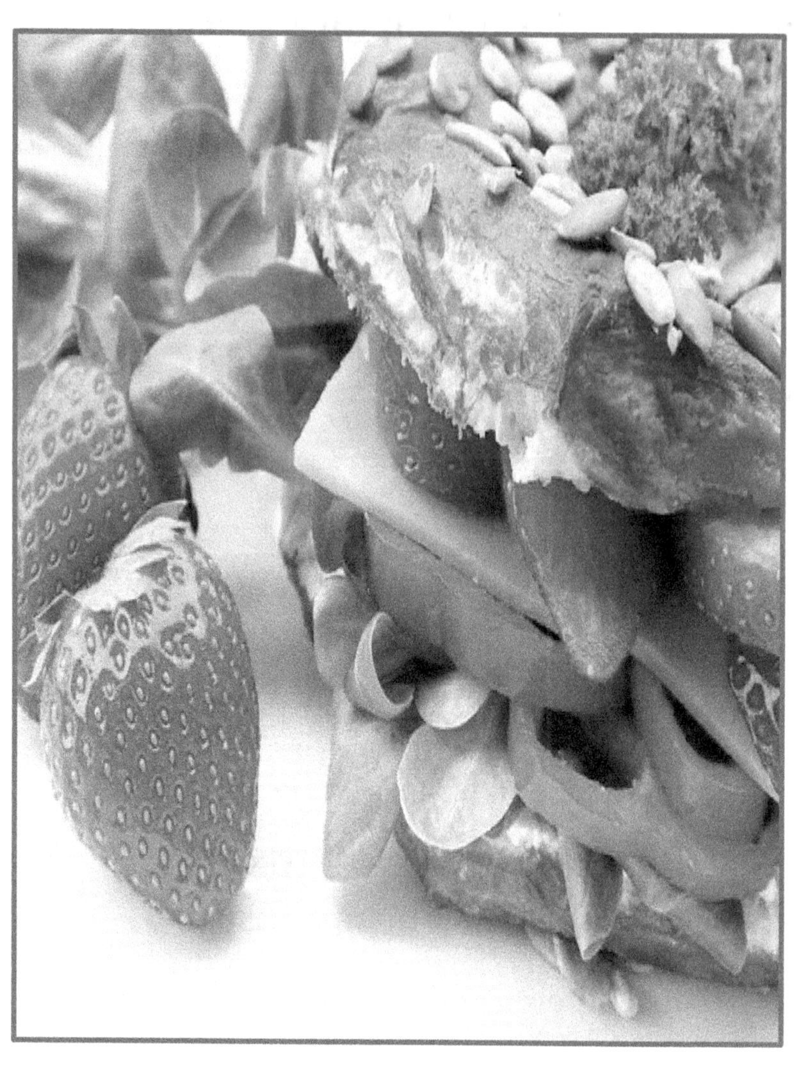

PART 8: HOLIDAY AND SPECIAL OCCASION MEALS

When celebrating holidays and special occasions, it's important to enjoy delicious and festive meals while keeping your diabetes management goals in mind.

Herb Roasted Turkey Breast

A succulent and flavorful turkey breast seasoned with herbs, perfect for holiday dinners.

Ingredients:

- 1 whole turkey breast (about 4 5 pounds)
- 2 tablespoons olive oil
- 2 tablespoons fresh rosemary, chopped
- 2 tablespoons fresh thyme, chopped
- 2 cloves garlic, minced
- 1 lemon, cut into wedges
- Salt and black pepper to taste

Instructions:

1. Preheat oven to 375°F (190°C).

2. Rub the turkey breast with olive oil, rosemary, thyme, garlic, salt, and pepper.

3. Place the turkey breast on a roasting pan and squeeze lemon wedges over it. Place the wedges around the turkey in the pan.

4. Roast for 1.5 to 2 hours, or until the internal temperature reaches 165°F (74°C). Let rest before slicing.

Cauliflower Stuffing

A low carb alternative to traditional stuffing, made with cauliflower, vegetables, and herbs.

Ingredients:

- 1 large head of cauliflower, grated into "rice"
- 2 tablespoons olive oil
- 1 cup diced celery

- 1 cup diced onions
- 1/2 cup diced carrots
- 1/4 cup chopped fresh parsley
- 1/2 teaspoon dried sage
- 1/2 teaspoon dried thyme
- Salt and black pepper to taste

Instructions:

1. Heat olive oil in a large skillet over medium heat. Add celery, onions, and carrots, and cook until softened, about 5 7 minutes.
2. Add grated cauliflower, parsley, sage, thyme, salt, and pepper. Cook for an additional 10 minutes, stirring occasionally, until cauliflower is tender and flavors are combined.

Green Bean Almondine

A light and elegant green bean side dish with almonds and a touch of lemon.

Ingredients:

- 1 pound fresh green beans, trimmed
- 2 tablespoons olive oil
- 1/4 cup sliced almonds
- 2 cloves garlic, minced
- 1 tablespoon lemon juice
- Salt and black pepper to taste

Instructions:

1. Blanch green beans in boiling water for 2 3 minutes, then transfer to an ice bath to stop cooking. Drain well.

2. Heat olive oil in a skillet over medium heat. Add sliced almonds and cook until golden brown, about 2 minutes.

3. Add garlic and green beans to the skillet. Sauté for 5 minutes until beans are heated through. Stir in lemon juice and season with salt and pepper.

Pumpkin Spice Cheesecake

Pumpkin Spice Cheesecake is a creamy, decadent dessert with the comforting flavors of fall. This recipe combines the richness of cheesecake with the warm spices of pumpkin, making it a delightful treat that can be enjoyed while managing Type 2 diabetes.

Ingredients:

For the Crust:

- 1 cup almond flour
- 1/4 cup granulated erythritol or other sugar substitute
- 1/4 cup melted coconut oil or unsalted butter
- 1/2 teaspoon ground cinnamon

For the Cheesecake Filling:

- 16 oz (2 cups) cream cheese, softened

- 1 cup canned pumpkin puree (not pumpkin pie filling)
- 1/2 cup granulated erythritol or other sugar substitute
- 1/2 cup plain Greek yogurt (full fat or low fat)
- 3 large eggs
- 1 teaspoon vanilla extract
- 1 teaspoon ground cinnamon
- 1/2 teaspoon ground nutmeg
- 1/4 teaspoon ground ginger
- 1/4 teaspoon ground cloves

For the Topping (Optional):

- Whipped cream (sugar free or made with a sugar substitute)
- A sprinkle of cinnamon

Instructions: Preheat your oven to 350°F (175°C).

Prepare the Crust: In a medium bowl, combine the almond flour, erythritol, melted coconut oil, and ground cinnamon. Mix until well combined.

Press the mixture firmly into the bottom of a 9 inch spring form pan to form an even layer.

Bake the Crust: Bake the crust in the preheated oven for 10 minutes. Remove from the oven and let it cool while you prepare the filling.

Prepare the Cheesecake Filling: In a large bowl, beat the softened cream cheese until smooth. Add the pumpkin puree, erythritol, and Greek yogurt, and mix until well combined.

Add the eggs one at a time, mixing well after each addition. Stir in the vanilla extract, ground cinnamon, nutmeg, ginger, and cloves.

Mix until the batter is smooth and well combined.

Bake the Cheesecake: Pour the cheesecake filling over the prepared crust in the spring form pan.

Bake in the preheated oven for 45 50 minutes, or until the center is set and the edges are slightly puffed. The cheesecake will still jiggle slightly in the center.

Cool and Chill: Turn off the oven and leave the cheesecake in the oven with the door slightly ajar for 1 hour. This helps prevent cracking.

Remove from the oven and refrigerate for at least 4 hours or overnight to set.

Serve: Before serving, top with sugar free whipped cream and a sprinkle of cinnamon if desired.

Nutritional Information (per 1 slice, assuming 12 slices):

- Calories: 220
- Carbohydrates: 12g
- Protein: 8g
- Fat: 18g
- Fiber: 3g
- Sugars: 5g

Tips:

- To prevent cracks in the cheesecake, ensure all ingredients are at room temperature before mixing.
- If you prefer a smoother texture, you can blend the filling ingredients using a food processor or blender before pouring it into the pan.
- For an extra touch of flavor, you can add a few chopped pecans or walnuts to the crust mixture.

Roasted Brussels Sprouts with Balsamic Glaze

Roasted Brussels Sprouts with Balsamic Glaze is a flavorful and nutritious side dish that brings out the natural sweetness of Brussels sprouts while adding a tangy touch with a balsamic glaze. This recipe is perfect for adding a healthy and delicious option to your meals, especially for those managing Type 2 diabetes.

Ingredients:

- 1 pound Brussels sprouts, trimmed and halved
- 2 tablespoons olive oil
- Salt and black pepper to taste
- 1/4 cup balsamic vinegar
- 1 tablespoon honey or a sugar substitute suitable for cooking
- 1 teaspoon Dijon mustard (optional)

- 2 tablespoons chopped fresh parsley (for garnish, optional)

Instructions:

Preheat your oven to 400°F (200°C).

Prepare the Brussels Sprouts: In a large bowl, toss the halved Brussels sprouts with olive oil, salt, and black pepper until evenly coated.

Roast the Brussels Sprouts: Spread the Brussels sprouts in a single layer on a baking sheet. Roast in the preheated oven for 2025 minutes, or until the Brussels sprouts are golden brown and crispy on the edges. Toss halfway through the cooking time for even roasting.

Prepare the Balsamic Glaze: While the Brussels sprouts are roasting, in a small saucepan, combine the balsamic vinegar and honey (or sugar substitute). Bring to a simmer over medium heat, stirring occasionally.

Let the mixture cook for about 57 minutes, or until it has reduced by about half and has a syrupy consistency. Stir in the Dijon mustard if using, then remove from heat.

Finish and Serve: Once the Brussels sprouts are roasted, transfer them to a serving dish. Drizzle with the balsamic glaze and toss to coat.

Garnish with chopped fresh parsley if desired. Serve warm.

Nutritional Information (per 1/2 cup serving):

- Calories: 130
- Carbohydrates: 12g
- Protein: 4g
- Fat: 8g
- Fiber: 4g

- Sugars: 6g

Tips:

For extra flavor, you can sprinkle some toasted pine nuts or chopped walnuts over the Brussels sprouts before serving.

Adjust the sweetness of the glaze by modifying the amount of honey or sugar substitute based on your taste preferences and dietary needs.

This dish can be prepared ahead of time and reheated in the oven to maintain its crispy texture.

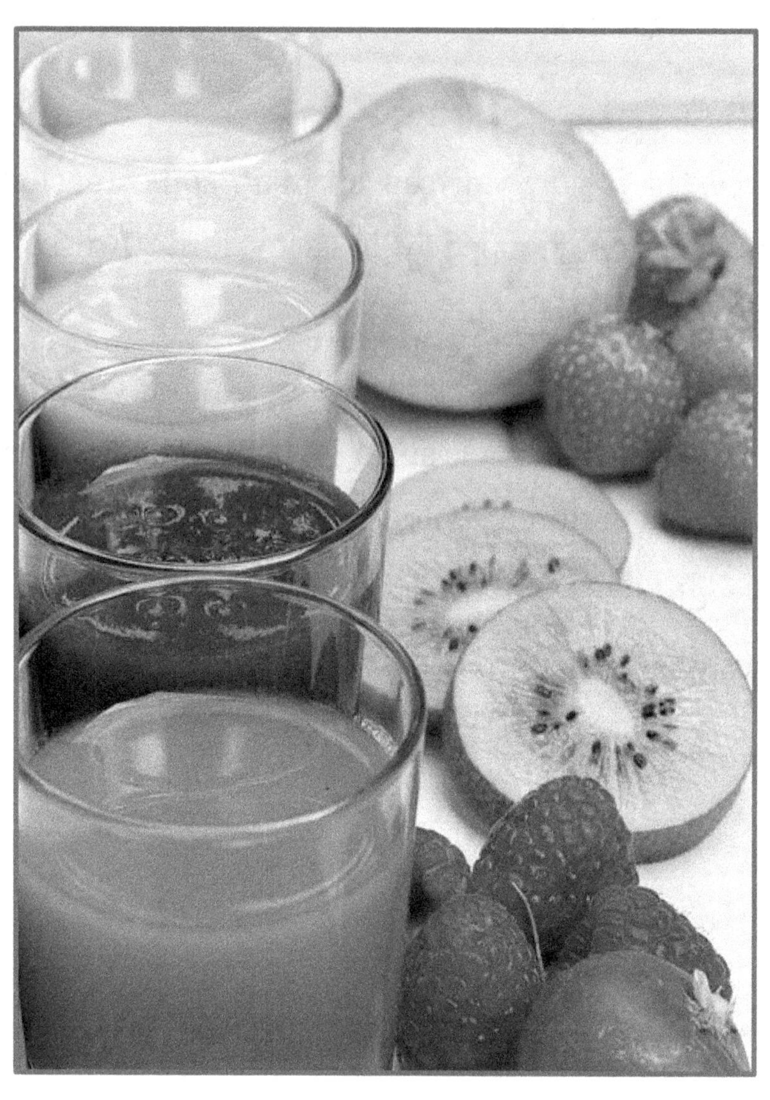

PART 9: TIPS AND TRICKS FOR LONG TERM SUCCESS

Maintaining a healthy lifestyle while managing Type 2 diabetes requires consistent effort and smart strategies. Here are some practical tips and tricks to help you achieve long term success in managing your diabetes and leading a healthier life.

Plan Your Meals

Create a Weekly Menu: Plan your meals and snacks for the week to ensure you have balanced, diabetes friendly options available. This helps you avoid last minute unhealthy choices.

Prepare in Advance: Cook and freeze meals in advance or prepare ingredients for quick assembly. This saves time and ensures you have healthy options readily available.

Balance Your Plate

Incorporate Lean Proteins: Include sources of lean protein such as chicken, fish, tofu, and legumes in your meals to help with blood sugar control and satiety.

Load Up on Vegetables: Aim to fill half your plate with no starchy vegetables. They are low in calories and carbs but high in fiber and nutrients.

Choose Whole Grains: Opt for whole grains like quinoa, brown rice, and whole wheat bread instead of refined grains. They have a lower glycemic index and provide more fiber.

Monitor Portion Sizes

Use Smaller Plates: Eating from smaller plates can help control portion sizes and prevent overeating.

Practice Mindful Eating: Pay attention to hunger and fullness cues. Eating slowly and savoring each bite can prevent overeating and improve digestion.

Stay Hydrated

Drink Plenty of Water: Aim for at least 8 glasses of water a day. Staying hydrated helps regulate blood sugar levels and supports overall health.

Limit Sugary Drinks: Avoid sugary beverages like soda and sweetened juices. Opt for water, herbal teas, or sparkling water with a splash of lemon or lime.

Stay Active

Incorporate Regular Exercise: Aim for at least 150 minutes of moderate intensity exercise per week, such as brisk walking, swimming, or cycling.

Find Activities You Enjoy: Choose physical activities that you find enjoyable to make it easier to stick with your routine. This could include dancing, gardening, or playing sports.

Monitor Your Blood Sugar

Track Your Levels: Regularly check your blood sugar levels as recommended by your healthcare provider. This helps you understand how different foods and activities affect your glucose levels.

Adjust as Needed: Based on your blood sugar readings, adjust your diet, exercise, or medications as advised by your healthcare provider.

Manage Stress

Practice Stress Reduction Techniques: Engage in activities like meditation, deep breathing, or yoga to manage stress. Chronic stress can impact blood sugar levels.

Make Time for Relaxation: Ensure you have time for hobbies and activities you enjoy, which can help reduce overall stress levels.

Seek Support

Join a Support Group: Connect with others who have Type 2 diabetes for shared experiences, encouragement, and tips. Support groups can provide valuable emotional support and practical advice.

Consult a Dietitian: Work with a registered dietitian or nutritionist who specializes in diabetes management to create a personalized meal plan and address any dietary concerns.

Stay Informed

Educate Yourself: Stay informed about diabetes management and treatment options. Knowledge helps you make better decisions about your health.

Keep Up with Research: Follow credible sources and updates on diabetes research and advancements to stay current with new information and strategies.

Set Realistic Goals

Set Achievable Goals: Break your long-term health goals into smaller, manageable steps. Celebrate your progress and stay motivated by recognizing your achievements.

Adjust as Needed: Be flexible and adjust your goals and strategies based on your experiences and any changes in your health status.

CONCLUSION

Managing Type 2 diabetes is a journey that demands a thoughtful and sustained approach. Through the strategies and recipes outlined in this book, you have the tools and knowledge to take charge of your health and make empowered choices.

Commitment to Your Health

Maintaining a diabetes friendly lifestyle involves more than just dietary changes; it encompasses a holistic approach to managing your condition. The key is to make gradual, sustainable adjustments that fit your lifestyle and preferences. From understanding how to balance your plate and monitor your portions to incorporating regular physical activity and managing stress, every small step contributes to a healthier you.

Celebrating Successes and Embracing Challenges

As you embark on this journey, celebrate each milestone, whether it's a successful meal plan, a new exercise routine, or improvements in your blood sugar levels. Recognize that there may be challenges along the way, but each challenge is an opportunity to learn and grow. Adapt your strategies as needed and continue to seek support and resources.

Looking Forward

The goal is not just to manage diabetes but to thrive despite it. By consistently applying the tips and recipes provided in this book, you can enhance your quality of life and achieve long-term health. Remember, you are not alone on this journey. Reach out to healthcare professionals, join support groups, and stay informed about the latest research and strategies.

Final Thoughts

Your journey with Type 2 diabetes is unique to you, and your path to success will be shaped by your personal choices and experiences. Embrace the principles of balanced nutrition, regular activity, and mindful living to create a sustainable and fulfilling approach to diabetes management. With persistence and dedication, you can achieve your health goals and enjoy a vibrant, healthy life.

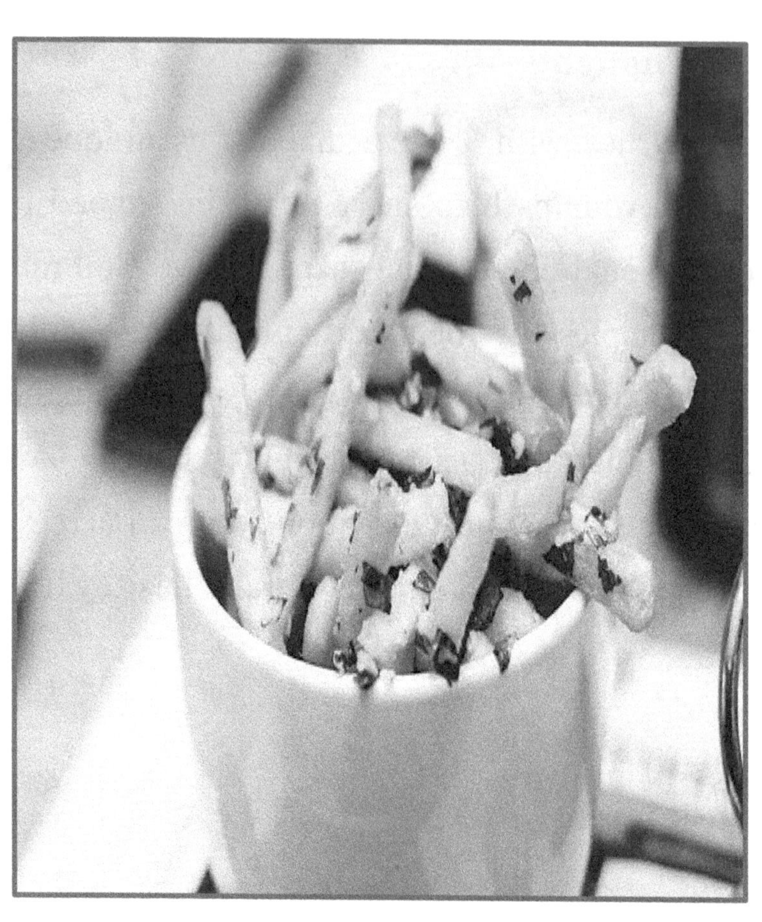

WE VALUE YOUR FEEDBACK

Thank you for choosing our cookbook, "Type 2 Diabetes Cookbook for Beginners: Naturally Control Blood Sugar and Achieve an A1C Below 5.7% Simple, Delicious Recipes for Reclaiming Your Health." We hope that the recipes, tips, and resources provided have been helpful in your journey toward better health.

Your feedback is important to us!

If you found this book useful, we would greatly appreciate it if you could take a moment to leave a review. Your insights help us improve and assist others in finding the right resources for managing Type 2 diabetes.

Please consider sharing your thoughts on:

How the recipes and tips have impacted your diabetes management.

Any specific recipes or sections that you particularly enjoyed.

Suggestions for future editions or additional content you would find helpful.

Where to Leave a Review: Online Retailers: If you purchased the book from an online retailer, you can leave a review on their website.

Social Media: Share your experience on social media and tag us, so we can see and share your feedback.

Thank you once again for your support. We wish you continued success and health on your journey